Dr Germain MANZEKELE BIN KITOKO

Vascular accidents: everyone's business?

Dr Germain MANZEKELE BIN KITOKO

Vascular accidents: everyone's business?

The challenge of family caregivers in Kinshasa

ScienciaScripts

This book is a translation from the original published under ISBN 978-620-6-71514-6.

Publisher:
Sciencia Scripts
is a trademark of
Dodo Books Indian Ocean Ltd. and OmniScriptum S.R.L publishing group

120 High Road, East Finchley, London, N2 9ED, United Kingdom
Str. Armeneasca 28/1, office 1, Chisinau MD-2012, Republic of Moldova, Europe
Printed at: see last page
ISBN: 978-620-7-97722-2

DEDICATION

I dedicate this work to an exceptional caregiver, Julie KATEMBO, who made me fully experience what it means to be a caregiver and spouse in the difficult moments at the end of her partner's life. Her dedication and strength have left a deep impression on me. As a healthcare professional, family member and caregiver, it was an unforgettable experience. **In memory of Raphael PALUKU KAHUMWIRE, who died in Paris on 12/13/2023, I would like to highlight the courage and tenacity of his wife Julie, who showed unfailing determination in the face of adversity. Julie** *showed remarkable resilience and infinite compassion throughout this ordeal. Her comforting presence and unconditional support were invaluable to the entire family. She handled every aspect of the situation with admirable strength and determination. Her love and devotion were palpable right up to her soulmate's last breath. Julie was a pillar of strength and support for Raphael, perfectly embodying the ideal of the dedicated caregiver. Her determination, kindness and generosity were an inspiration to all those around her. Through her example, Julie reminds us of the importance of compassion, unconditional love and unwavering support in the face of life's trials. Her courage and determination were pillars to lean on in the darkest moments. Her unwavering commitment to overcoming obstacles was not only remarkable, but inspiring to all who had the privilege of knowing her. Julie found within herself an unshakeable strength, one that led her to face every ordeal with courage and resilience. Her ability to remain steadfast in the face of adversity was a lesson to us all, reminding us that nothing is insurmountable with determination and compassion. Her positive attitude and unconditional support were key elements in the fight against Raphael's illness. As a dedicated caregiver, she devoted every waking moment to watching over him, providing loving care and giving him all the love he needed. Through her example, Julie shows us how the power of love can be an engine of healing and resilience. In this time of grief, we will always remember Julie as a rock, a source of light and hope in the most difficult of times. Her boundless devotion and infinite* *compassion will remain etched in our memories for all eternity. Rest in peace Raphael and Julie courage!*

Dr MANZEKELE BIN KITOKO Germain

ACKNOWLEDGEMENTS

I'd like to express my gratitude to all my trainers, my elders, my peers and fellow fighters.

I pay tribute today to the great Professor S. MAMPUNZA for his emerituship, trying to find the right words to express how decisive his influence has been in my scientific career. It is thanks to him that I am here, having accepted to guide me as a true academic mentor.

I would also like to thank Prof. MPEMBI Nkosi Magloire for his inspiration, advice and support throughout this work, not forgetting Prof. MANANGA LELO, Prof. MATONDA, Prof. BANZULU BOMBA, Prof. KASWA, Prof. Adélard N'SITU MANKUBU, Prof. NGOMA MALANDA and the entire CNPP team, as well as the heads of the psychiatry and neurology departments.

I'd like to express my gratitude to all my trainers, my peers and my fellow fighters.

Honor and gratitude bmy dear wife Rose Lyliane Rose AMANI MAKULUKYO and our children Marielle MASIKA MANZEKELE and Christelle KAVIRA MANZEKELE, for their invaluable support and sacrifices.

My parents KAMBALE MANZEKELE and KAHINDO VAKOLAVATI, my sisters FURAHA MANZEKELE, ANNE MANZEKELE, FAZILA MANZEKELE KATUNGU MANZEKELE Riziki and my brother Azor MUKWAMI also deserve my gratitude. I would also like to pay special tribute to my mother, the model woman Marie Jeanne KAHINDO VAKOLAVATI, who is celebrating 50 years in the profession. I admire her faultless career. She is an inexhaustible source of inspiration, love, patience and perseverance. As a courageous and combative nurse, she embodies the quintessence of strength and resilience. My mother is an example of determination and professional success, and I am extremely proud of her longevity and unwavering commitment. Mom, you are not only an exceptional mother figure, but also a fearless and combative nurse. Thank you, Mom.

I am immensely grateful to Mr Benoit KISUKI, his family, Mr Kakule Makulukyo Kahundu Alfred my father-in-law, my in-laws for their unfailing support. Their kind gestures will remain forever engraved in my heart. I would also like to pay tribute to my mentor, the late Dr Ferdinand BAHIMBIRANA PALUKU, and to my late mother-in-law, KAHONGYA JEANNE MBAGHENDA. I hope they can see from the hereafter that this work is a real source of pride for them.

TABLE OF CONTENTS

LIST OF ABBREVIATIONS, ACRONYMS AND SYMBOLS

AF : Family caregiver

ANAES: Agence Nationale d'Accréditation et d'Evaluation en Santé (French National Agency for Health Accreditation and Evaluation)

STROKE : Cerebral Vascular Accident

ADL: Activities of Daily Living

CH: Hospital Center

CHU: Centre Hospitalier Universitaire

CNSA: Caisse Nationale de Solidarité pour l'Autonomie)

CRPH K: Centre de Rééducation des Personnes Handicapées de Kinshasa (Kinshasa Rehabilitation Center for the Disabled)

 PADV: Post Stroke Depression

HADS: Hospital Anxiety and Depression Scale

HSA: Health Savings Account

INRB: Institut National des Recherches Biomédicales m

RS: modified Rankin Scale

WHO: World Health Organization

 PAF: Loss of Functional Autonomy

PHQ-9: Patient Health Questionnaire

DRC: Democratic Republic of Congo

ADD: Anxiety-Depressive Disorder

UNIKIN: University of Kinshasa

UNV: Neurovascular Unit

ZBI: Zarit Burden Inventory

Caregivers are truly unsung heroes, juggling the emotional and physical challenges of caring for a sick loved one. The notion of burden is not enough to describe the complexity of their situation. Firstly, their workload is extremely heavy, with an average of 8 hours a day devoted to essential tasks such as grooming, dressing, meals and medication. This reality generates stress and anxiety that can have a serious impact on their physical and mental health.

Secondly, the caregiver's personality plays a decisive role in how he or she experiences the situation. Some see it as a sacred duty, while others feel constrained. This vision will inevitably influence the way they manage their workload.

Finally, several factors intensify the pressure on family caregivers, such as depression, feelings of anger, perceived lack of social support, or the burden of isolation as a primary caregiver.

It is crucial to recognize and support these caregivers, as their well-being directly impacts the quality of life of the sick people they care for. Caregivers are true unsung heroes, masterfully juggling the emotional and physical challenges of caring for a sick loved one. The mere idea of "burden" is not enough to describe the complexity of their situation. Finally, there are many factors that add to the pressure on family caregivers, such as depression, anger, lack of perceived social support or isolation as the primary caregiver. It is essential to recognize and support these caregivers, as their well-being has a direct impact on the quality of life of the sick people they care for. To alleviate their emotional burden, it is crucial to promote their well-being by encouraging social support, regular breaks, stress management and help-seeking. In addition, education and information about their loved one's illness can help caregivers feel better prepared and more confident. In cases of psychological burden, it is also important to consult a mental health professional for help. As each situation is unique, it's crucial that family caregivers find strategies that work for them to preserve their health and mental equilibrium.

To relieve their psychological burden, it's essential to promote their well-being. Encouraging social support, regular breaks, stress management and help-seeking are key strategies to help them get through this difficult period while preserving their health and mental equilibrium.

SUMMARY

Introduction:

In stroke patients, there is a solid literature on the psychological burden of family caregivers. In the DRC, no such study has been conducted among caregivers of stroke survivors. The aim of this study is to describe the emotional workload of these caregivers in Kinshasa.

Method:

In this descriptive study, 85 "caregiver/patient" dyads were recruited at the Centre de Rééducation des Personnes Handicapées de Kinshasa by stroke patients. ZBI and HADS assessments were carried out to evaluate caregivers' psychological burden and severity. Fischer's exact test was used to correlate psychological burden with qualitative variables, and Mann Whitney's U test to compare means of quantitative variables.

Results:

The majority of family carers (84.7%) expressed a feeling of work burden. This burden was severe in a third of caregivers. Depression and anxiety were experienced by 35% and 33% of family caregivers, and by just under 31% and 27% of patients. Burden was associated with anxiety and depressive disorders in the caregiver-patient dyad and with the patient's degree of disability.

Conclusion:

For the majority of family carers, accompanying loved ones with stroke in Kinshasa was a burden. Because of the severity of this burden, caregivers were more depressed and anxious than patients. Burden was related to caregiver depression, anxiety and anxiety-depressive disorder, as well as anxiety-depressive disorder and disability severity.

Key words: *Psychological burden, family caregivers, stroke, depression, anxiety, Kinshasa.*

Chapter 1. INTRODUCTION

1.1. CHOICE AND INTEREST OF SUBJECT

Stroke is the third leading cause of death, the second leading cause of dementia and the leading cause of acquired disability in adults in Western countries (8,34,46,72). In sub-Saharan Africa, stroke ranks third in terms of mortality and motor disability, with alarming statistics: 45% of neurology admissions in Dakar and 32.9% in Lomé are due to stroke (8), while in the DRC (54), stroke accounts for 6% of all cases in Kinshasa. However, these data remain fragmentary due to the absence of surveys of the general population. According to the WHO, 15 million people are affected by stroke every year, resulting in 5 million deaths and 5 million permanent disabilities (8). This burden weighs heavily on families and communities, and is one of the major challenges facing healthcare systems in developing countries, alongside heart disease (8). Despite considerable progress in diagnosis and treatment, stroke remains a major public health problem due to its frequency, severity and cost. Around half of all stroke survivors become dependent, with tragic consequences for their physical, mental, family and professional lives (63). Complete recovery from stroke remains rare, with 75% of survivors suffering lasting after-effects, 33% becoming dependent for life, and 25% never returning to work (89). Every minute counts in stroke, as it is equivalent to the loss of 2 million neurons (89). With the right treatment and prompt care, it is possible to reduce the after-effects and significantly improve patients' quality of life. The impact of stroke-related sequelae varies, depending on the nature of the stroke and the speed with which it is managed (63). Stroke is a diagnostic and therapeutic emergency requiring early management (39). In France, for example, thrombolysis could be useful for 15% of stroke patients. However, only 1% receive this treatment.

1.2. ISSUES

In Africa, family members are often responsible for supporting the elderly, the frail and/or disabled, and people of all ages suffering from chronic illness (stroke and its consequences). However, supporting a loved one often entails consequences for the family carer, such as impacts on his or her financial situation, career, social situation or health (48,49,84,86). It is essential to recognize and support family carers in order to maintain and/or improve their quality of life, as well as that of the people they care for. This promotes the status of family carers and improves the quality of support. According to recommendations for good practice istroke care, it is recommended that the family and family carer be involved at all levels of care (8). These recommendations suggest more dynamic screening, assessment and monitoring of the needs and coping levels of patients, families and caregivers. The use of this comprehensive patient-centred approach offers more positive outcomes in terms of recovery and adaptation after stroke (44,62). Indeed, once at home, stroke survivors are cared for by their families. Family members and caregivers are faced with responsibilities and tasks that sometimes require necessary knowledge and skills. This situation creates a burden for caregivers. Bocquet and Andrieu (14) have defined burden as "all the physical, psychological, emotional, social and financial consequences that the caregiver undergoes". The burden that falls on caregivers is sometimes heavy and frequently leads to depression, with rates as high as 60% (48,49).

But caregivers who report a high workload risk disrupting their personal lives and their role as patient support (45). When caregivers' psychological difficulties go undetected and untreated, they can lead bfamily tensions and acts of abuse, and even to a decline in the satisfaction of patients' needs and activity levels (45). For around twenty years, international studies have focused on the importance of informal caregivers. However, despite the strong interest shown by researchers, there is little data in this field in sub-Saharan Africa. In the DRC, no studies have been carried out, although Mpembi has highlighted the importance of including the psychosocial component in the overall care process for stroke patients in Kinshasa (61).

1.3. OBJECTIVES

1.3.1. General

Encourage improved stroke management by addressing the psychopathological problems of family carers.

1.3.2. Specific

• Assessing the frequency of perceived burden in family caregivers of patients after stroke;

• Identifying the severity of perceived burden in family caregivers of stroke survivors;

• Identify elements related to the psychological burden of family caregivers.

Chapter 2. GENERAL

2.1. DEFINITIONS OF CONCEPTS

2.1.1. Family or natural caregiver

A family caregiver can be defined as "the non-professional person who provides assistance on a principal basis, in whole or in part, to a dependent person in his or her entourage, for the activities of daily life. This regular assistance may be provided on a permanent or non-permanent basis, and can take many forms, including: nursing, care, support with education and social life, administrative tasks, coordination, constant vigilance, psychological support, communication, domestic activities, etc." (44,48).

2.1.2. Burden

a) Definition

Burden is defined as the physical, psychological, emotional, social and financial consequences borne by the caregiver (48, 52). It is the result of an imbalance between the constraints and possibilities of the family caregiver.

b) History and consequences for the caregiver

The concept of "Burden" began to emerge in the 1980s, with a series of studies analyzing the impact of caregivers' daily tasks on their physical and mental health. These studies showed that caregivers tended to neglect their own health. Indeed, some had put forward the hypothesis that stress could have biological consequences for caregivers, such as immune response disorders and hyper-cortisolaemia (48, 52).

The impact of caregiving on health is well documented. Depression is thought to affect 30% of caregivers (68). Other disorders include anxiety, fatigue, social isolation and feelings of helplessness or guilt (48, 49).

Nevertheless, the caregiver's role can have positive consequences in terms of mental well-being. Some say that taking care of their loved one has enabled them to acquire tolerance, strength of character and patience (48,52).

Initially, some researchers based on stress and coping theory saw caring for a loved one as work to which the same diagnosis could be applied as for professional stress: exhaustion and burn out (48,52).

Recent research emphasizes the socio-affective dimension. They approach the subject by focusing on the nature of the caregiver-care receiver relationship. In this context, family ties and the quality of the relationship between the two subjects influence the caregiver's state of health and stress (63).

Dependency raises questions about everyone's role within the family. The major risk is that of infantilizing the dependent person. The caregiver feels obliged to take charge of his or her relative's household, and assumes the role of the person in charge. This feeling of responsibility makes the caregiver "their parent's parent".
Indeed, the results of several studies have shown that caregivers generally did not wish to give up their profession. They were, however, often forced to reduce their working hours. This results in a loss of earnings.

2.1.3. Types of assistance

The duty of loyalty and the role of the eldest child in providing for his or her parents are all invisible mechanisms that play a part in the caregiver's choice of involvement, whether consciously or unconsciously. Helping experiences can be divided into four categories.

2.1.3.1. Alteration aid

It focuses on the negative aspects of the help provided. This type of help leads to a feeling of great exhaustion.

2.1.3.2. Commitment aid

In this type of assistance, the caregivers' attention is very high. Nevertheless, they manage tgive meaning to their investment. It's a response to the unconscious desire to pay off the family debt.

2.1.3.3. Fear helper and satisfaction helper

In both cases, the notion of duty comes into play:

- In the first case, there is no notion of self-realization. It's simply a question of responding to the needs of a loved one by carrying out tasks that are deemed to be burdensome.

- In the second case, caregivers are able to find meaning in their help, and may find it rewarding. In this case, stress does not seem to have a major hold on caregivers.

2.1.4. Activity

It is the performance of a task or action for an individual. In terms of activities, restrictions are difficulties in performing certain tasks.

Activities of daily living (ADLs) involve basic personal care
These include feeding oneself, washing and showering, looking after one's appearance, walking, getting up from a chair and using the toilet.

2.1.5. Rehabilitation

It's the restoration of a disabled person's optimal functional, physical and psychological autonomy.

2.1.6. Recovery

This is the process by which a person recovers the body's structure, functions, activities and participation (without any time limit).

2.1.7. Leave

This is the service that enables patients to leave hospital earlier than usual, thanks to the support provided by structured interdisciplinary teams during the hospitalization period and the first few weeks at home. Rapid supported discharge modifies the conventional clinical pathway to offer more acceptable services to patients undergoing rehabilitation.

2.1.8. Cerebrovascular accident

The World Health Organization (WHO) defines stroke as "the rapid development of localized or global clinical signs of cerebral dysfunction with symptoms lasting more than 24 hours, which can lead to death without any apparent cause other than a vascular origin" (61).

2.2. MODEL OF A PATIENT'S JOURNEY THROUGH THE CARE OF A VC

Lindsay et al, Canadian Best Practice Stroke Strategy. This model emphasizes the role and responsibility of healthcare providers at each stage of the continuum of stroke care. The patient and family benefit from active participation in recovery and open communication with the healthcare team. The patient's social reintegration is the major step where all actions converge.

2.2.1. Transition

It's the movement of patients between locations, providers, objectives and various healthcare settings.

2.2.2. Support for transitions

2.2.2.1. Objective of transition management

Facilitate a smooth transition across the continuum of care and provide support to the patient, family and caregivers. This transition enables the family system to sustainably achieve an optimal level of adaptation, as well as good health outcomes and quality of life after stroke. The physical, emotional, environmental, financial and social factors that influence the process need to be taken into account.

Working with patients, families and caregivers to design and implement a transitions plan that sets goals is flexible enough to respond to changing needs as they evolve.

Successful transition management requires close collaboration between healthcare professionals, the patient, family and caregivers. It encompasses the organization, coordination, education and communication required during the process by which the patient, family and caregivers move from one stage and setting of care to another: acute care, recovery, reintegration, adaptation and end-of-life care.

2.2.2.2. Support

For patients and their families, it's the provision of care and services and referral to available resources to meet the needs of the patient, family and caregivers throughout the stroke recovery process, from a variety of perspectives.

The goal of patient, family and caregiver support is to provide everyone with the tools and information they need to take charge of their own or a loved one's recovery from stroke, and to maximize participation and fulfillment in life roles. Support must take into account special needs, coping mechanisms, strengths, difficulties and the home situation.

2.2.2.3. Case manager/stroke care system pilot

The system pilot or case manager is often a social worker or a professional in a related field. He or she is often involved in the acute care phase and provides follow-up care for the first six months after a stroke, depending on the needs of the patient and family. An important role of the system pilot or case manager is to provide emotional support to the patient, family and caregivers, as well as help with the practical aspects of post-stroke adaptation (63).

The system pilot or case manager works closely with healthcare professionals, social workers, volunteers and providers. He or she is also responsible for personalized patient, family and caregiver education.

2.3. CARE FOR CAREGIVERS

It goes hand in hand with that of patients.

2.3.1. Psycho-education

Patient, family and caregiver education should include information, self-management skills, and training for family and caregivers to help them participate in stroke management and provide safe care.

It will focus on the following objectives: fostering decision-making about care and recovery, encouraging self-management in patients, families and caregivers after stroke. Patient education should emphasize empowerment, such as activity planning, role models, problem-solving and decision-making strategies, reinterpretation of symptoms, identification of risks in relation to current and ideal lifestyle, and the level of risk the patient wishes to accept to maintain or improve health after stroke (e.g., decisions about smoking, diet, blood pressure management). Key topics of self-management training include physical activity, symptom and risk factor management techniques, secondary stroke prevention, nutrition, fatigue and sleep management, medication use, coping with fear, anger and depression, cognitive and memory changes, training in communication with healthcare professionals and related disciplines, problem-solving and health decision-making. Family and caregiver education should include training in self-care techniques, communication strategies and physical handling techniques, food preparation and modifications for patients with dysphagia. It will also incorporate the self-management model to encourage patients to try as much as possible to perform tasks without the help of others. Other objectives will address preferences for activities of daily living, access to community services and resources, and problem-solving techniques. Orientation within the healthcare system should be organized. However, with the patient's permission, family and caregivers should be invited and encouraged to take part in treatment sessions with the patient and have their questions answered. Family and caregivers need to be taught certain patient care skills, and given opportunities for practice and feedback to ensure safe care for both them and the patient (e.g., bed-to-chair transfers, feeding techniques, positioning of the hemiplegic limb). Learning and training in the basics of moving and holding, and facilitating daily activities, reduces burden, anxiety and depression, and helps to improve caregivers' quality of life and satisfaction over a three- to 12-month period. Moreover, patients whose caregivers have undergone training report a good quality of life and psychological state for 3 to 12 months (58).

2.3.2. Improved support

Some caregivers need more support from family and professionals to manage the responsibilities inherent in their caring role. Through this intervention, the caregiver can clarify the support he or she needs and envisage the right care.

2.3.3. Information and orientation

The caregiver receives information on potential solutions and different support services. The information provided must address existing and emerging concerns. The better informed the caregiver, the easier it is to make decisions and prepare for the future.

2.3.4. Psychotherapy

Caregiver distress can often be alleviated by psychotherapeutic intervention. Marriot et al. demonstrated the effectiveness of a 14-session psychotherapeutic program for distressed family caregivers in reducing depressive symptoms and burden by working on the caregiver's feelings and coping methods (52). Cognitive-behavioural approaches appear to be particularly useful when caregivers have unrealistic ideas.

2.3.5. Discussion groups

The benefits vary. Some caregivers have divergent and unclear agreements. This is why the psychologist will play an important role in assessing caregivers' needs and identifying those who will benefit from specific intervention.

2.3.6. Accommodation for caregivers

According to ANAES, this is a temporary home, a kind of respite care facility as exists for Alzheimer's caregivers in industrialized countries. The accommodation will enable the caregiver to go away without fearing for his or her loved one. Specialized teams will take care of the patient, enabling the caregiver to have some time to himself or herself.

Chapter 3: MATERIAL AND METHODS

3.1. FRAME

The Kinshasa Rehabilitation Center for the Physically Handicapped was selected for this study because it is the only rehabilitation center with the staff and equipment required to care for most physically handicapped patients. The center's various activities are organized into three departments (medical, administrative and financial, technical and social). The medical department includes various services such as consultation, hospitalization, as well as the physiotherapy department comprising the adult neurology, child neurology and physiotherapy units, and the orthopedics and traumatology departments.

3.2. NATURE AND PERIOD OF STUDY Type of study

This descriptive study was conducted at the rehabilitation center for disabled people in Kinshasa between December 2014 and September 2015.

3.3. POPULATION STUDY

Family caregivers and stroke patients followed up at the Kinshasa rehabilitation center for the physically disabled, who agreed to take part in the study, formed the convenience sample of 85 patient-caregiver dyads.

3.4. DATA COLLECTION

Data collection was carried out by two interviewers. They were familiar with the research protocol and trained to carry out various assessment tests. They were responsible for supervising, explaining or assisting caregivers or patients who were unable to complete the self-evaluation tests on their own. The patients' level of autonomy was assessed using the modified Rankin scale.

3.5. INCLUSION CRITERIA Caregiver

- Primary caregiver (same place of residence as patient)

- 18 years of age or older,

Patient

- Documented survivor of a non-aphasic stroke (CT scan of the brain, see the center's registry)
- Be 18 years of age or older
- Understand the questionnaire

3.6. EXCLUSION CRITERIA

Caregiver

- Qualified healthcare professional
- No history of behavioral disorders or substance abuse

Patient

- Aphasia
- Cognitive disorders and dementia
- Behavioral disorder

3.7. CONSIDERATION ETHICS

In order to take part in this study, written consent was obtained from the patient and their primary caregiver. Participants were given a thorough and informed explanation of the study's objectives, the method of assessment and safety. Confidentiality was assured. The patient-caregiver dyad had the option of terminating their participation in the research at any time during the study for personal reasons. The Ethics Committee of the University of Kinshasa validated the protocol.

3.8. DATA COLLECTION TOOLS

3.8.1. Zarit Burden Iventory (ZBI)

The Zarit Burden Inventory was developed to assess the burdens faced by healthcare professionals in caring for patients with dementia. In this study, caregivers were asked about each of the 22 items on this scale. Caregivers were asked to identify when they felt a particular emotion in their caregiving relationship. The frequency could vary from 0 "never", 1 "rarely", 2 "sometimes", 3 "quite often" to 4 "almost always". The sum of the scores for each item gives an overall score, which can theoretically fluctuate from 0 to 88.

The perceived burden is greater as the score increases: the burden is light between 21 and 40, moderate between 41 and 60, and severe above 61.

3.8.2. HADS (Hospital Anxiety and Depression Scale)

The Depression Anxiety Scale (Zigmond and Snaith HADS) was used to assess depression and anxiety. It comprises 14 items rated from 0 to 3;

of which seven questions relate to anxiety (total A) and seven to depression (total D), resulting in two scores (maximum score for each =21). According to Zigmond and Snaith (55), the criteria for two sub-scores to identify cases with symptoms of depression or anxiety are as follows:

- 0 to 7: no anxiety or depression

- 8 to 10: anxiety or depression suspected

- 11 to 14: anxiety or depression

- 15 to 21: severe anxiety or depression

According to Ibbotson et al (55), the thresholds for the overall score are :

- 0 to 14: absence of anxiety-depressive disorders

- 15 to 42: existence of anxiety-depressive disorders

In our study, a HADS score above 7 was associated with depression or anxiety, while depression or anxiety was considered mild for a score of 8 to 10, moderate for a score of 11 to 14 and severe for a score of 15 to 21.

3.8.3.   Rankin scale

The Rankin Scale was developed in 1957 to assess the effects of stroke and was improved in 1988 to make it more practical. Since then, the modified version, or MRS, has been used to assess disability after stroke. The Rankin Score is designed to assess functional autonomy, taking into account WHO elements such as body function, activity and participation.

The use of this scale enables disability to be assessed in a less restrictive and less costly way. Data can be collected from patients by telephone or mail, without the need for a further patient visit. This can be extremely captivating for epidemiological research involving large populations. The Rankin indicator ranges from 0 to 6:

-    A score of 0 indicates that the patient shows no signs of disability.

-    A score of 1: no significant handicap, despite symptoms, patient able to perform all usual tasks and activities.

-    A score of 2: slight incapacity, patient unable to perform all tasks, but able to devote himself to his occupations without assistance.

-    A score of 3: moderate disability, requiring some assistance, but the patient can walk alone.

-    A score of 4: moderate disability, inability to walk without assistance and inability to manage bodily needs without assistance.

-    A score of 5: severely disabled, bedridden patient requiring continuous care and monitoring.

-    A score of 6 indicates death.

According to neurologists, all patients with a score of 3 or more are considered to have a severe disability.

3.9. DATA COLLECTION PROCEDURE

Potential participants were identified by Rehabilitation Center experts during their follow-up interview. If a client (caregiver-patient dyad) was interested in participating in the research, it was necessary to obtain written informed consent. The client was informed of the details and objectives of the study, and could stop participating at any time. During the patient's care, the family caregiver completed the burden scale (ZBI), as well as the depression and anxiety scales. The patient then completed the depression scale. The Rankin score was assessed by observing the patient walking and performing rehabilitation exercises.

3.10. ANALYSIS OF DATA

Data were analyzed using SPSS 22 software. Results were presented in the form of frequency tables for categorical variables and means for quantitative data. The association between different categorical variables was examined using Fischer's exact test. To compare means, we used the Mann-Whitney U test. The statistical significance level chosen was 5%. The following variables were dichotomized: perceived burden, depression or anxiety and degree of patient disability. Two groups were chosen for burden: "presence of burden" for Zarit scores above 20, and "absence of burden" for Zarit scores below 20.

"For anxiety and depressive disorders, a score above For anxiety or depressive disorders, a score greater than 7 indicated the presence of disorders, while a score less than or equal to 7 indicated their absence. The presence of anxiety and depressive disorders was associated with an overall score greater than 14, while a score less than or equal to 14 was considered absent. A Rankin score greater than 2 was perceived as a severe disability, while a score less than or equal to 2 was considered less severe.

Chapter 4: RESULTS

In this study, 85 caregiver-patient dyads were assessed and interviewed. The results of our study were published in scientific article: ***"Psychological Burden in Stroke Survivors and Caregivers Dyads at the Rehabilitation Center of Kinshasa (Democratic Republic of Congo): A Cross-Sectional Study"***.

4.1. SOCIO-DEMOGRAPHIC CHARACTERISTICS

Table 1. Socio-demographic characteristics of family carers

VariableN 85	n (%) or mean ± SD
Age (years)	42,3±14,339
Gender	
Female58	(68.2)
Male27	(31.8)
Civil status	
Married	49 (57,6
Other	36 (42,4
Education level	
No	4 (4,7
Primary	14 (16,5
Secondary	32 (37,6
College or university	35 (41,2
Jobs	
Non	31 (36,5)
Yes54	(63.5)

The caregivers, with an average age of 42 ± 14, were mainly women, married, employed and with a high school or university degree.

Table 2. Socio-demographic characteristics of patients

Variable	N85 n (%) or mean ± SD
Age (years)	59,02±13,08
Gender	
Male	45 (52,9)
Female	40 (47,1)
Diploma obtained	
No	27 (31,8)
Primary	10 (11,8)
Secondary	16 (18,8)
Graduates and more	32 (37,6)
Jobs	
Assets	54 (63,5)
Other	31 (36,5)

The patients, whose mean age was 59 ±13 years, were predominantly male (52.9%), professionally active and well educated (university or high school graduates).

4.2. CHARACTERISTICS OF THE CAREGIVER'S RELATIONSHIP WITH THE PATIENT

Table 3. Helping relationship variables

Variable	N85 n (%) or mean ± SD
PAF	
mRS	
Average score	2,588±1,2
Yes	43 (50.6)
Non	42 (49.4)
Patient relations	
Spouse	32 (37,6)
Son/daughter/grandchild	35 (41,2)
Brother/sister/cousin	9 (10,6)
Uncle/aunt	3 (3,5)
Other	6 (7,1)
Previous experience as a caregiver No	56 (65,9)
Yes	29 (34,1)
Caregiver information No	72 (84,7)
Yes	13 (15,3)
Caregiver training Yes	7 (8,2)
No	78 (91,8)
Motivation	
Family help	78 (91,8)
Other	7 (8,2)
Caregiver support	
Non	81 (95.3)
Yes	4 (4,7)
Duration of assistance (years)	1,691 ±1,338

The majority of FAs were from the patient's family, 65.9% of whom were first-time caregivers. Children or grandchildren accounted for 41.2%, followed by spouses with 37.6%. Functional disability was observed in 50.6% of patients. Of the 10

FAs, 8 received no social support, training or information, and their main motivation was to participate in family solidarity.

4.3. PSYCHOMETRIC PROFILES

Table 4. Psychometric profile of family caregivers

Variables	N 85 n (%) or mean ± SD
Anxiety	
Yes	28 (32,9)
No	57 (67,1)
Average score	5,85±3,856
Depression	
Yes	30 (35,3)
No	55 (64,7)
Average score	6,15±4,385
TAD	
YES	28 (32,9)
No	57 (67,1)
Average score	11,88±7,12
ZBI	
21-88 (Burden)	72 (84,7)
21-40 (Light to moderate)	55 (64,7)
41-60 (Moderate to severe)	16 (18,8)
Average score	30,17±10,81

Burden was expressed by 84.7% of family caregivers, of whom 64% expressed a mild to moderate burden, 18.8% a moderate to severe burden and 1.2% a severe burden. The FAs presented respectively 35.3% depression, 32.9% anxiety and 31.8% anxiety-depressive disorders.

Table 5. Psychometric profile of patients

Variables	n (%) or mean ± SD
Depression	
Yes	27 (31,8)
No	58 (68,2)
Average score	5,64±3,89
Anxiety	
Yes	21 (24,7)
No	64 (75,3)
Average score	4,86±3,688
TAD	
Yes	23 (27,1)
No	57 (72,9)
Average score	10,56±6,417

The incidence of depression is 31.8%, while anxiety is 24.7% and both anxiety and depressive disorders are 27.1%.

Table 6. Caregiver variables and perceived burden

Variables	Burden present N 72 (%) or avg ±	Burden absent N 13 (%) or avg ± SD	P
Age (years)	42,75±14,081	40,38±16,148	0,467ψ
Gender			0,465*
Male	24(33,33)	3(23,07)	
Feminine Employment	48(66,67)	10(76,93)	
Assets			0,086*
	43(59,72)	11(84,61)	
Other diploma obtained	29(40,28)	2(15,39)	
Secondary and higher			0,726*
	56(77,78)	11(84,62)	
Other	16(22,22)	2(15,38)	
Civil status			1,00*
Married	41(56 ,94)	8(61,54)	
Other Relationship	31(43,06)	5(38,46)	
Spouse			0,758*
	28(38,89)	4(30,77)	
Other	44(61,11)	9(69,23)	
Caregiver experience			0,720*
Yes	24(33,33)	5(38,46)	
No Training	48(66,67)	8(61,54)	
Yes			0,992*
	11(15,28)	2(15,38)	
No	61(84,72)	11(84,62)	
Information			0,938*
Yes	6(8,33)	1(7,69)	
No Support	66(91,67)	12(92,31)	
Yes			0,581*
	3(4,17)	1(7,69)	
No	69(95,83)	12(92,31)	
Anxiety	6,21±3,911	3,85±2,911	0,0027ψ
Depression	6,78±4,237	2,69±3,614	<0,001ψ
TAD	12,99±6,943	6,54±4,977	0,001ψ
Duration of assistance	1,1583±1,408	1,2285±1,26436	0,995ψ

Ψ :U Mann Whitney, * : Fisher test

Burden was strongly related to depression (p = <0.001), anxiety (p = 0.0027) and the caregiver's anxiety-depressive disorder (p = 0.001). Caregiver burden was not statistically related to caregiver age, relationship to the patient, level of education, duration of support, employment, motivation, support or gender.

Table 7. Patient variables and FA burden

Variables	Present burden N 72 (%) or Moy±ET	No burden N 13 (%) or Moy±ET	p
Age (years)	59,92 ±13,593	54,08 ±10,727	0,127 ψ
Gender			0,367*
Male	40(55,56)	5(38,46)	
Female	32(44,44)	8(61,54)	
Jobs			0,212*
Assets	48(66,67)	6(46,15)	
Other	24(33,33)	7(53,85)	
Anxiety	5,11±3,668	3,46±3,479	0,097ψ
Depression	5,93±4,043	4,00±3,367	0,077ψ
TAD	11,13±6,404	7,46±5,768	0,038ψ
PAF mRS	2,74±1,151	1,77±1,166	0,007ψ

Ψ :U Mann Whitney, * : Fisher test

Caregiver burden was related to the presence of anxiety-depressive disorder (p=0.038) and to the severity of the patient's disability (p=0.007). Severity of burden was not related to the survivor's age, gender, anxiety or depression, level of education or employment.

Chapter 5. DISCUSSION

The aim of this study was to analyze the considerable impact of the burden on family members caring for stroke patients, as well as the intensity of this burden for caregivers of stroke survivors. In addition, it sought to determine the various elements that contribute to the emotional burden of family members involved in caregiving. The originality of this study lies in the fact that it took place after the initial phase of the stroke, thus enabling a more in-depth and relevant analysis of the situation of family caregivers.

5.1. SOCIO-DEMOGRAPHIC CHARACTERISTICS OF THE CAREGIVER AND VARIABLES IN THE HELP RELATIONSHIP

6.1.1. Age

The average age of FAs was 42.39 years (σ =14), around seventeen years older than patients. In India, the average age of caregivers was 45.6 years, some 22 years younger than that of patients (13). By contrast, in Luxembourg, Barbara and colleagues found that the average age of caregivers was 59.1 years, 5 years younger than her patient (9). The average age of caregivers probably differs according to life expectancy in each country. In the Congo context, this is the age of the adults practicing their profession. For this reason, support has a significant financial impact on the household (65). Stroke has disastrous consequences not only for individuals, but also for society, due to its cost and the loss of earnings it can generate, both for the patient and for the carer, when the latter was a salaried employee.

5.1.2. Gender

Most family carers are women, accounting for 68.2%. This trend is observed in almost all studies, with varying proportions. According to Selim Omrani, there are 2 women for every 1 man among family caregivers (78). Analyzing 20 articles on family caregivers of stroke patients published between 1986 and 1998, Beth et al.

found that 60 to 100

% of caregivers were women, wives or daughters of the survivor (14). However, Qurat's survey in Pakistan contrasts with this trend, with 70% of caregivers being men (73). Indeed, the division of care and support tasks for people who have suffered a stroke can be influenced by prevailing social norms and gender expectations. For example, in some cultures, women are traditionally perceived as the primary caregivers within the family, which may explain why they are more often the primary caregivers for stroke patients in some regions. Conversely, men may take on this role in societies where gender expectations give men a more pre-eminent status in caring for family members. Female gender and culture could be factors contributing to the burden of FAs. In the Democratic Republic of Congo, female FAs are frequently exhausted and have to reconcile their domestic duties, work and patient care. As a result, female FAs face a high risk of psychological suffering and additional stress, which explains the high prevalence of depressive disorders, anxiety and anxiety-depressive disorders among female caregivers. Balhara has demonstrated that gender can be used to predict anxiety in FA (7).

5.1.3.   Civil status

The majority of FAs were married, representing 57.647%. This is in line with findings in other countries. According to Barbara and colleagues' study in Luxembourg, 85.4% of stroke patients were married (9). Barbara also shows that the role of patient carer always seems to be an extension of the traditional role of woman, wife or mother, even if she has other social responsibilities (16). In reality, it seems that the psychosocial effects of stroke affect women more than men, for a woman who will have to reconcile her domestic work with her patient-care responsibilities. The psychosocial consequences of stroke are likely to affect women more than men, as it is the woman who will have to reconcile her domestic work with her responsibilities as patient carer.

5.1.4. Jobs

Among caregivers, 63.5% were employed. The risk of psychological suffering is higher when the caregiver is responsible for the family's financial resources. In addition to the burden of caring tasks, FAs were faced with a budget deficit. Caring for a loved one who has survived a stroke has an impact on their work and generates a loss of income. Sometimes, the FA is forced to take time off, reorganize their schedules or even resign. According to the CNSA's 2011 activity report, April 2012, 47% of those providing assistance to patients were employed or apprenticed. For 36%, helping relatives had a negative impact on their career, and 26% of those who were working or had already worked had taken time off (74). Only 15% changed their work schedule, of which 65% changed their working hours and 36% reduced them (74).

5.1.5. Education level

More often than not, family caregivers had a high level of secondary (37.6%) and university (41.2%) education. This finding is comparable to that found in studies (Mpembi) (61, 67). In Poland, on the other hand, caregivers' level of education was lower than in our series, with 34% at secondary level and 13% at university level (49). In the Congolese context, access to rewarding employment is generally linked to educational level. Caregivers belong to a privileged category, whether they are employees, managers or employers. They face considerable stress, making them more vulnerable to psychological distress and weight.

5.1.6. Helping experience

The majority (65%) of FAs were first-time helpers. The sudden onset of stroke is a thunderclap for the family, causing considerable upheaval - six times out of ten, as Michèle Baumann reports (10). Studies show that many caregivers lack knowledge about stroke, which can increase their sense of burden. For example, 22.1% of caregivers of dependent patients do not know enough about stroke (68). The gaps relate to prevention, risk factors, stroke sequelae, recovery, prevention of recurrence and necessary environmental adaptations (68). The gap between caregivers' abilities to provide care and patients' health needs could lead to caregiver burden. Without prior preparation for this role, caregivers pay a heavy price. They are torn between understanding the stroke crisis, the hope of recovery and the exit crisis. It's all happening so fast that caregivers are under considerable stress. These inexperienced caregivers don't even have time to develop appropriate coping mechanisms, and are quickly exhausted (11). Many caregivers feel the need for further training. Questions asked by caregivers on the Internet help to identify their needs. Online forums have provided answers. Main themes include managing emotions, financial impact and fear of the future (68). Other themes addressed include the balance between personal life and the role of caregiver, the relationship between caregiver and cared-for, and relations with healthcare professionals (68).

5.1.7.   Motivation

Family caregivers were mainly motivated by the idea of contributing to family solidarity (80%). According to Gosman Hedstrôm and his team, caregivers provide valuable help to their spouses, regardless of the severity of the initial stroke (38). This behavior is in line with African tradition, where the individual is defined by his or her membership of a community or family. This belonging manifests itself in involvement at critical moments such as a serious illness or important events like a wedding. Although help is often motivated by feelings towards sick loved ones, most caregivers find themselves in this role imposed by circumstances (86). Some experience this responsibility as a constraint, increasing the risk of decompensation and exhaustion. Within families, it is not always clear how caregivers are designated. A survey in France revealed that 4 out of 10 caregivers feel constrained for economic reasons. Their motivation is fuelled by various feelings: family duty, a strong emotional bond with the sick person, a sense of usefulness, and fear that someone else will take less care of their loved one (35).

5.1.8. Social support

Some 95.3% of family caregivers (FCs) said they had not received any social support from their loved ones. This result may seem surprising, but it can be explained by the nature of stroke, which is a pathology characterized by different phases. Initially, during the crisis, family support is generally strong, but gradually weakens as hope of recovery diminishes and isolation sets in. Our study was conducted at an advanced stage of the disease, which explains why a large number of FAs reported a lack of support. Another possible explanation is that primary caregivers do not fully recognize the help provided by other family members. Indeed, it is rare to find a single caregiver in African families. Family members involved in home care contribute indirectly to supporting the patient. It is therefore important that the primary caregiver assigns them specific tasks to optimize their support, so that they can concentrate on the patient's more complex care. In studies on the phenomenological analysis of the experiences of Family Caregivers (FC), it is clear that these people feel abandoned when it comes to economic support (84,86), especially in developing countries such as the Democratic Republic of Congo, where health policies do not provide financial compensation for caregivers, leaving them to bear the costs of care alone. The most crucial social support for them is undoubtedly financial assistance for the patient's care. Research by Andrew et al. reveals that 21% of carers suffer from a lack of support, while 54% express the need for some respite, but only 24% manage to get it (68). Clearly, financial support is crucial, as a third of caregivers are seeing their income fall, while half are seeing an increase in personal expenses (44). Indeed, employed carers contribute more financially and are less involved in day-to-day tasks (44). On the other hand, they remain active in other aspects, such as care coordination, household chores and administrative assistance (44).

5.2. BURDEN FELT BY CAREGIVERS

In 84.7% of cases, family carers experienced a burden, a percentage almost identical to that found in a study carried out in Nigeria (83.5%). According to Rigby H et al., between 25% and 54% of caregivers consider their role to be a real burden, a perception that could be explained by the marked differences in socio-economic realities and healthcare systems between countries (75). This underlines the universal nature of the challenges faced by caregivers, whether in France or elsewhere in the world. Compared with industrialized nations, caregivers in developing countries have less financial support and resources to care for their loved ones. Indeed, the burden felt by family carers varies according to the country and its level of development. Caregivers in developing countries appear to be more affected by this burden, perhaps due to socio-economic factors such as lack of resources, financial support and adequate healthcare facilities. In the Democratic Republic of Congo, families have to bear the cost of care alone, placing an additional burden on caregivers. Caregivers' investment in care affects their quality of life, sometimes forcing them to reduce their working hours or resign. Around 90% of carers see their lives change after an accident affecting their loved one. These figures highlight the heavy responsibility placed on the shoulders of these dedicated people, who often sacrifice their own well-being to care fotheir loved ones. It is crucial to recognize and support the essential role of family carers, in order to prevent burnout and ensure their mental and physical health.

5.3. DEPRESSION, ANXIETY AND ANXIETY-DEPRESSIVE DISORDER (ADD)

5.3.1. Caregiver depression

The percentage of people with depressive symptoms among family carers was 35.3%. This figure is close to the results of the study by Rigby and his team, where the prevalence of depression ranged from 39 to 52% (75). In China, the study conducted by W. TANG and his team revealed an alarming rate of emotional distress among family carers, reaching between 52 and 55% (85). According to the study by Qurat and his team, carers often experience greater psychological distress than their relatives (73). These findings highlight the intense psychological pressure placed on these relatives who provide support and care for dependent people, and the imperative need to provide appropriate support and resources to prevent mental and emotional exhaustion among caregivers who devote themselves unstintingly (89). Indeed, family carers show symptoms of depression and anxiety, reflecting the considerable emotional burden they carry. The results of our study corroborate this reality. Congolese family caregivers experience depressive and anxiety disorders due to the heavy emotional burden they carry. Our results highlighted the reality of vulnerability and high rates of depression among Congolese family caregivers, who are often left alone and without support to manage their responsibilities. The work of Choi Kwon and his team also highlighted the persistence of this problem at all stages of stroke (22). Lena Olai and colleagues have highlighted the negative impact of caregiver depression on patient rehabilitation, underlining the importance of providing adequate support to caregivers (58).

5.3.2.   Caregiver anxiety

The anxiety rate among caregivers is 32.9%, higher than that of stroke patients (19, 23) and the general population (53). This can compromise the quality of their support and jeopardize their helping relationship. This finding raises concerns about the often neglected mental health of caregivers, who are forced to juggle their own well-being with that of their loved one requiring care. Caregivers' anxiety compounds their burden and creates a vicious circle. This constant fear prevents them from taking time for themselves and affects their ability to provide effective help, further increasing the caregiver's burden. According to Balhara, this dynamic creates a spiral where the patient's anxiety reinforces that of the caregiver and vice versa, creating a cycle that is difficult to break (7). Specific support and training programs should be put in place to help them manage their anxiety and strengthen their resilience. Supporting caregivers can also help improve the quality of care provided to stroke patients, by fostering a stronger, more effective helping relationship. Support systems such as discussion groups and stress management training are needed to prevent caregiver burnout and ensure quality support. Growing concerns about caregivers' mental health underpin the need to provide them with adequate support to prevent any deterioration in their psychological well-being. Specific support and training programs should be put in place to help them manage their anxiety and strengthen their resilience.

5.3.3. TAD for caregivers

Almost a third of people caring for stroke patients at home actually suffer from anxiety-depressive disorders (32.9%). Despite this, international research on the subject is scarce. Family carers, exhausted by the stress of managing care at home, may find themselves confronted with anxiety or depressive disorders. Lack of rest, worries about the patient's health and financial difficulties can exacerbate these problems (45, 86). It is crucial to identify these disorders in caregivers in order to offer them appropriate treatment and prevent any deterioration in their well-being. There is evidence that lack of support and training for carers can lead thigh levels of psychological distress (68). Indeed, unprepared carers in the Democratic Republic of Congo are often faced with delicate and complex situations that they do not know how to handle, which can lead them to develop anxiety-depressive disorders. Moreover, the lack of recognition of their role and needs can also contribute to the onset of these disorders (68). Caregivers, who are often taken for granted, lack the resources and support they need to cope with the emotional and physical burden of their role. The situation is all the more worrying in the Congolese context, where the lack of training plunges caregivers into psychological distress. Caring for patients and performing complex nursing procedures without adequate training can be extremely stressful, leading to anxiety and depression (84,

86). The lack of recognition and support only exacerbates the situation for these caregivers, leaving them to face a monumental task alone (68). Family caregivers (FCs) face physical and emotional challenges when caring for stroke patients at home. They face high levels of stress and anxiety due to lack of time to rest, the need to constantly monitor the patient, deteriorating health, advanced age, fear of stroke recurrence or even death (84, 86). In addition, FAs' nervousness and stress may be exacerbated by economic problems and excessive workload (84,86). Studies have shown that spousal carers are particularly prone to depression due to role reversal in their daily tasks (86). It is crucial to identify these disorders in FAs in order to provide them with adequate support, avoid overload and prevent deterioration in the helping relationship. It is imperative to make healthcare professionals and family carers aware of the risks to which they are exposed, in order to implement appropriate support and accompaniment measures. By early detection of signs of anxiety and depression in family carers, it is possible to introduce therapeutic interventions and psychological support programs to prevent a deterioration in their mental well-being. Caring for these caregivers not only promotes their own health, but also the well-being of the patients they care for.

5.4. BURDEN, CAREGIVER AND THE HELPING RELATIONSHIP

Family caregivers play a key role in the recovery of stroke patients, providing both physical and psychosocial support. However, there is an imbalance between caregivers' skills in providing care and patients' health needs, which can result in emotional burden for caregivers. Caregivers caring for stroke patients at home are more likely to suffer from anxiety and depressive disorders (86). The constant stress associated with caring for these patients can have a negative impact on caregivers' mental health, affecting their quality of life and ability to provide quality care (45, 86). Indeed, family carers of people who have had a stroke experience a deterioration in their quality of life, neglect of their own health, a reduction in their professional and leisure activities, as well as psychological suffering marked by feelings of isolation, loneliness and uncertainty (68, 84, 86).

Caregivers are reported to have high levels of anxiety and depression. Caregivers face a mountain of challenges that go far beyond the day-to-day tasks of providing assistance. In addition to the psychological repercussions, their burden translates into an increased risk of mortality and physical illness (45). Most caregivers reported feeling this burden significantly, manifesting as symptoms such as depression, anxiety and anxiety-depressive disorder. Surprisingly, these disorders seemed to affect family carers more than the people they were helping. Research by Olai Kotila also highlighted similar findings, revealing that the burden felt by patients and their loved ones was just as profound (58). The degree of burden felt would largely depend on the patient's and caregiver's ability to adapt to their situation. Those who are able to accept the reality of their situation more quickly generally show less distress than those who struggle to adapt. Caregivers themselves experience high levels of anxiety and depression, in addition to increased risks of somatic illness and mortality. These repercussions can even lead to a breakdown in the care provided, jeopardizing the health of the patients being cared for. The results of a meta-analysis of 22 studies and nearly 3,000 caregivers, followed for at least one month after the onset of stroke in their loved one, revealed that certain patient-specific variables had a significant impact on caregiver burden (45). These included impairments in daily activities and high anxiety levels, while other factors such as gender (predominantly female), neurological deficits and depression had a less marked effect (45). Similarly, caregiver-specific aspects such as depression and anxiety are also key factors in this equation (45). With regard to caregivers, significant effects were observed in depression and anxiety (45). Factors such as the gender of the caregiver, the type of relationship with the patient, physical health status and professional situation also had more or less pronounced consequences on the burden felt, with a small to moderate effect size (45). Clearly, the role of caregiver can be extremely demanding, with serious repercussions, both physically and psychologically. In a study by Denno et al. which examined anxiety and depression in caregivers of patients with spasticity, 21.6% of caregivers were found to suffer from anxiety, and 22.2% were diagnosed with a depressive syndrome (29). Their survey revealed that over half the caregivers (55.6%) had experienced depressive symptoms in the two weeks prior to the study, and almost 10% reported a particular severity of these symptoms (29). These findings corroborate those of Sennfält et al. who identified a low level of psychological well-being affecting up to 51.4% of caregivers (68). There was also an increase in negative emotions such as frustration, fatigue, anxiety and sadness among caregivers, depending on the degree of dependence of their loved one (68). In addition, this study highlights that caregivers' physical health is also more vulnerable than that of the general population (68). It is crucial to consider that some caregivers may be more fragile due to their own health problems or advanced age (48). In Poland, Jaracz and colleagues demonstrated that caregivers' emotional suffering was actually due to the help they provided to the patient. These authors studied the prevalence of burden in caregivers of stroke patients after 6 months and 5 years (48). At 6 months, 44% of caregivers reported experiencing considerable burden, and this figure remained stable at 30% at 5 years (48). The main factors contributing to this burden were time spent monitoring the loved one, anxiety and poor ability to manage stress, which were also present at 5 years, in addition to the extent of the loved one's disability (48). These also suggested interventions to improve caregivers' management skills

(49). Kamel and his team in Jordan reported that caregivers

experienced high levels of depression and burden (52). Denno and his team showed that anxiety and depression were correlated with increased caregiver burden (29). Caregivers experienced 55.3% PHQ-9 depression and 21.6% anxiety (29). Research by Saban's team at Loyola University Chicago revealed high levels of stress associated with poor biological response, confirmed by cortisol levels, in the wives of stroke patients (77). These findings have led some researchers to define the "contagious effect" of stroke psychopathology in the families of patients and their carers. Because of its prolonged duration, stroke provokes physical and psychological dependency and a restructuring of roles within the family, where the carer (or close family) is often more affected than the patient, and left to fend for himself. In the DRC, the lack of support programs for caregivers makes them extremely vulnerable to the physical, psychological and other consequences associated with their status. It's a real biopsychosocial tragedy.

5.5 SOCIO-DEMOGRAPHIC CHARACTERISTICS OF PATIENTS

5.5.1.   Age

The average age of stroke patients in the Democratic Republic of Congo is 59.02 years, which is lower than the average for industrialized countries. A recent study in Nigeria revealed an average age of 59 among the study population, confirming results already observed in other studies carried out in sub-Saharan Africa (68). Sagui noted an average age range of 44.5 to 61 years, suggesting that the majority of strokes occur in this age group (31). It would therefore appear that the 50s and 60s are critical periods in terms of stroke risk, which is vital information for prevention and healthcare in sub-Saharan countries. This result can be explained by the short life expectancy in these countries, leading to an early occurrence of these accidents.

5.5.2 Gender

Men slightly outnumbered women in our study group (52.9% vs. 47.1%). The majority of studies favoured a male preponderance, with a ratio of between 1.3 and 1.5, as women would benefit from the protective effects of estrogen on the vessels before the menopause (61). After the menopause, a rebalancing is likely, bringing the proportions back to equality.

5.5.3.   Education level

The patients' level of education was high. This suggests that stroke mainly affects individuals who are potentially civil servants or salaried employees in the various sectors of the country's socio-economic life. Stroke therefore impacts the active socio-economic class and hinders the country's production and socio-economic development. It is a real obstacle to socio-economic progress (61).

5.5.4.   Jobs

In 63.5% of cases, patients claimed to have worked up to the time of stroke. This result corroborates the findings of Mpembi, who found that 64% of patients were involved in their work (61). Balhara, even reported a high risk of suicide among caregivers whose patients were the main providers of funds (7). Stroke mainly affects the working population, representing a financial catastrophe for families, the community and society in general.

5.6. PATIENT DEPRESSION, ANXIETY AND TAD

5.6.1.   Depression

CVAD was present in 31.8% of patients. Zahiruddin othman et al. reported a 32% prevalence of depression in patients (91). Mpembi et al. observed a 21.40% prevalence of depression in patients (61). The prevalence of post-stroke depression varies between studies, ranging from 21.40% to 32% (91,68). Factors such as patient characteristics and the diagnostic criteria used influence these results. For example, a study in Lagos found that 25% of patients were depressed (69). Furthermore, 22.9% of stroke survivors were diagnosed with depression, mainly moderate to severe (69). Post-stroke depression is associated with high healthcare costs, significant post-stroke disability and reduced quality of life (68).

5.6.2.   Anxiety

According to our study, nearly a quarter of stroke patients suffer from anxiety. In Burkina Faso, the prevalence of this disorder also amounted to almost a third of patients, or 27.8% (23). These figures contrast with the average of 18% obtained through clinical interviews, and 25% through psychometric assessments (19). International data show that anxiety persists over time, affecting around 20% of patients in the first month after stroke, then 23% between 1 and 5 months, and finally 24% after 6 months (19). However, a study by Mpembi shows a lower proportion, with only 10% of patients affected by post-stroke anxiety (61). This wide variation in the prevalence of anxiety in stroke survivors highlights the influence of cultural, social, individual and methodological factors. The impact of anxiety on patient recovery is significant, affecting quality of life, motivation to undergo treatment and ability to participate in rehabilitation activities.

5.6.3. TAD

Anxiety-depressive disorders (ADD) have been found in 27.1% of stroke patients. However, there is a lack of in-depth studies on this subject. Researchers often tend to examine these disorders individually, without taking into account the fact that they can occur together and have common causes in the same patient. It is important to consider these disorders in a hierarchical order, from anxiety to depression to anxiety-depressive disorder. Factors contributing to these disorders include loss of self-confidence, social isolation, role changes, job loss and disturbance of self-image (84,86).

5.7. CAREGIVER AND PATIENT BURDEN

In our study, burden was strongly correlated with the severity of the patient's disability. This correlation is found in numerous studies (91).

In Poland, Jaracz and colleagues obtained similar results (48). A patient suffering from severe dependence will require the constant presence of a caregiver and more consistent care. The time devoted to care and the complexity of care in such a situation increase the caregiver's burden and affect his or her professional and leisure activities. In addition, caregivers of patients in a situation of high dependency find it difficult to accept their loved one's situation (84,86). Caregiver burden was strongly associated with the presence of anxiety and depressive disorders in the patient. The presence of anxiety-depressive disorders also leads to an increase in the caregiver's caregiving time, and would result in further deterioration of the helping relationship by reinforcing the constraining and complex activities associated with certain symptoms of these disorders, such as abulia, apathy, hopelessness and feelings of worthlessness or of being a burden to others (84,86). This can lead bconflict and mistreatment of patients by their caregivers. Caregivers with little knowledge of the onset of such complications may perceive them as "whims". When the caregiver is confronted with emotional problems, and when the patient is more dependent and also suffering from an emotional disorder, the caregiver experiences an increased burden. This illustrates the downward spiral in the helping relationship that occurs when caregivers are left to their own devices. According to various authors, overburdened FAs will be unable to meet their social demands, especially when the survivor has severe physical limitations (40). This overload may be compounded by a lack of support from family members. As highlighted by Good Practice in Stroke Care, managing the mental health of post-stroke patients is essential to improving their quality of life and promoting recovery. By integrating the psychological dimension into post-stroke care, it is possible to reduce the burden of depression and help survivors make a full recovery.

Chapter 6. CONCLUSIONS AND OUTLOOK

Our research has shown that :

The person accompanying the stroke patient is often a younger woman, either a wife or a daughter.

In general, most caregivers face a moderate burden, but for 2% of them, the burden is heavy. Anxiety, depression or anxiety-depressive disorder are symptoms of caregiver burden severity.

Caregivers are more likely than patients to experience emotional difficulties.

Caregiver burden was influenced by the patient's functional incapacity and the patient's or caregiver's emotional difficulties. When the caregiver is confronted with emotional problems, and when the patient is more dependent and also suffering from an emotional disorder, the caregiver experiences an increased burden. This illustrates the downward spiral in the helping relationship that occurs when caregivers are left to their own devices.

OUTLOOK AND RECOMMENDATIONS

51

Outlook

Emotional problems are common among caregivers of stroke patients. These difficulties have a negative impact on the patient's rehabilitation process. Large-scale, multi-center studies are needed to take into account crucial parameters such as the personality profile of caregivers and patients, the nature of the pre-existing relationship between caregiver and patient prior to stroke, stress management mechanisms, the beneficial effects of caregiver assistance, and the temporal evolution of this relationship between caregiver and cared-for.

Recommendations

i.   Within the Ministry of Public Health, it is crucial to recognize the essential role of family caregivers as vital partners in the care of patients with chronic diseases, particularly stroke. They are key players in the day-to-day support and well-being of patients. It is imperative to organize awareness-raising and information campaigns aimed at the general public, to highlight the consequences for the health of those who accompany a sick loved one. It is crucial to highlight the importance of taking care of oneself as a caregiver, to avoid exhaustion and risks to one's own health.

ii.   Dear managers of the Centre de Rééducation Post- Hospitalisation (CRPH) de Kinshasa and dear care professionals. It is absolutely essential to include caregivers in the treatment of stroke patients. Their role is crucial to recovery and disease management. It is vital to provide them with clear information on the different treatment options available and the nature of the stroke. In addition, it is imperative to train family carers on how to help and what their responsibilities are. It is essential to carry out a thorough assessment of these caregivers to identify any mental pathology linked to their role, and to direct them towards appropriate care. In order to effectively support caregivers, it is strongly recommended that a liaison psychiatry team be set up within the facility, to ensure adequate psychological follow-up for caregivers, thus helping to improve the quality of life of stroke patients. Let's work together to ensure comprehensive, compassionate care for stroke patients, by actively and effectively integrating their carers into the therapeutic process.

work limits

This work encountered two major constraints. Firstly, the use of a scale that focused solely on the negative effects of the helping relationship, leaving out the beneficial aspects mentioned in the literature. Secondly, the exclusion of patients with behavioural disorders, aphasia and cognitive impairment limited our ability to fully assess the impact of caregiver burden in this category of patients. It is highly likely that this burden is actually heavier than our results suggest. The conclusions drawn from this study are based solely on the population studied, and it would therefore be wise to replicate this study by including more diversified samples in the future. In addition, an in-depth analysis of the caregivers' load profile and the various associated factors should be considered to assess their evolution over time.

BIBLIOGRAPHY

1.   Akosile CO, Okoye EC, Nwankwo MJ, Akosile CO, Mbada CE, Quality of life and its correlates in caregivers of stroke survivors from a Nigerian population. Qual Life Res. 2011 Nov; 20(9):1379-84. doi: 10.1007/s11136-011-9876-9. Epub 2011 Mar 6.

2.   Amelia Didier, the needs of families of cerebro-injured patients in the hospital environment

hospital rehabilitation july 2014

3.   Anderson, C.S., Linto, J., Stewart-Wynne, & E.G. (1995). A population-based assessment of the impact and burden of caregiving for long-term stroke survivors. Stroke, 26, 843849.

4.   Anne Forster,Lesley Brown,Jane Snrith,Allan House, Peter Knapp, John J Wright, John Young Information provision for Stroke patients and their caregivers. Cochrane Data base of systematic Reviews. 2012, 11 (2) CD001919.

5.   Anu Berg, Lic Psych; Heikki Paloma¨ki, MD; Jouko Lo¨nnqvist, MD;Matti Lehtihalmes,Lic Phil; Markku Kaste, MD Depression Among Caregivers of Stroke Survivors Stroke.2005;36:639-643

6.   Assogba Komi et al, Quality of life, anxiety and depression among stroke survivors in Togo African Journal of Neurological Sciences 2011-vol 30, N°1

7.   Balhara YP, Verma R, Sharma S, Mathur SA study of predictors of anxiety and depression among stroke patient-caregiversJ Midlife Health. 2012 Jan; 3(1):31-5. doi:
10.4103/0976-7800.98815.

8.   Balougou Agnon Ayelola,Koffi Grunitezk Eric K et al.Accidents vasculaires cérébraux chez le jeune (15 à 45ans) dans le service de neurologie du CHU Campus de Lome AJNS 2008Vol.27,N°2

9.   Barbara BUCKI, Elisabeth SPITZ, Michèle BAUMANN The esteem felt in

and its psychosocial determinants 2011

10. Baumann M, Briançon S, Deschamps JP. The family support network and the Heath Promotion. Arch. Public Health. 1992; 50:387-95.

11. Berg, A., Palomäki, H., Lönnqvist, J., Lehtihalmes, M., & Kaste, M. (2005). Depression among caregivers of stroke survivors. Stroke, 36, 639- 643.

12. Beth Han ,MA ,William E, Haley ,PhD, Family caregiving for Patients with Stroke Review and Analysis Stroke.1999,30, 1478-1485.

13. Bhattacharjee M, Vairale J, Gawali K, Dalal PMF, actorsaffecting burden on caregivers of stroke survivors: Population-based study in Mumbai (India). Ann Indian Acad Neurol. 2012 Apr; 15(2):113-9. doi: 10.4103/0972-2327.94994.

14. Bocquet H, Andrieu S (1999) " Le burden ": un indicateur spécifique pour les aidants familiaux.Gérontologie et Société,89,155-166.

15. Brodaty H., Green A., Koschera A., Meta-analysis of psychosocial interventions for caregivers of people with dementia, 2003

16. Bucki, Barbara, Elisabeth Spitz, and Michèle Baumann. "Caring for people after stroke: emotional reactions of male and female informal caregivers," Public Health, vol. 24, no. 2, 2012, pp. 143-156.

17. Calasanti T, King N. Taking "women's work" like a man: husbands' experiences of care work. Gerontologist. 2007; 47(4):516-27.

18. Caputo A., Study of the quality of life of post-stroke patients and their caregivers hospitalized in a stroke unit at the Annecy hospital, 2011.

19. Charlotte Cosin. Post-stroke mood disorders, characterization and early detection. Psychology and behavior. École pratique des hautes études - EPHE PARIS, 2016.
French. NNT:2016EPHE3051

20. Chau JP, Thompson DR, Chang AM, Woo J et al. Depression among Chinese stroke survivors six months after discharge from a rehabilitation hospital. J Clin Nurs. 2010 Nov; 19(21-22):3042-50. PubMed, Google Scholar 32.

21. Cheng HY, choir SY, Chau JP, The effectiviness of psycho social

interventions for stroke family caregivers and stroke survivors :a systematic review and meta-analysis Patient education and counselling 2014, 95 (1) ,30-44

22. Choi-Kwons S,Kim Hg,Kwon Su,Kin JS. Factors affecting the burden on caregivers of stroke survivors in South korea Arch.Phys ned Rechabil2005,86:1043-8

23. Christian Napon, Alfred Anselme Dabilgou, Alassane Dravé, Julie Marie Adelaide Kyelem, Jean Kaboré, Post-Stroke Anxiety in Hospitals in Burkina Faso

24. Claire Boutoleau, Fardeau de l'aidant dans la pathologie démentielle,

Psycho /Neuropsychiatrvieil/2009,7 special 15-20

25. Cohen C, Colantonio A,Vermich L(2002) Positive aspects of caregiving:rouding out the caregiver experience .International Journal of Geriatric Psychiatry,17,184-188.

26. Cossi Marie Joelle, Charge des Accidents Vasculaires Cérébraux (AVC) A Cotonou (Bénin), March 2012.

27. Dalal S, Beunza JJ, Volmink J, Adebamowo C, et al. Non- communicable diseases in sub-Saharan Africa: what we know now. Int J Epidemiol. 2011 Aug; 40(4):885-901. PubMed | Google Scholar

28. Deborah Jacks Camak MSN, RNC Nursing Instructor[*] Addressing the burden of stroke caregivers: a literature review 10 JUN 2015 DOI: 10.1111/ jocn. 12884.

29. Denno MS, Gillard PJ, Graham GD, DiBonaventura MD, Goren A, Varon SF, Zorowitz R. Anxiety and depression associated with caregiver burden in caregivers of stroke survivors with spasticity. Arch Phys Med Rehabil. 2013 Sep;94(9):1731-6. doi:

10.1016/j.apmr.2013.03.014. Epub 2013 Mar 30. PMID: 23548544.

30. Doan Q, Brashear A, Gillard P, et al. Relationship between disability and health-related quality of life and caregiver burden in patients with upper- limb poststroke spasticity. PM R 2012; 4:4-10.

doi: 10.1016/j.neurol.2017.01.168

31. E. Sagui, Strokes in Sub-Saharan Africa ,MedTrop2007 ,67 596_600, Handicaps-Incapacity-Dependence Survey 2004.

32. Eremand, Les motivations qui amènent à accompagner les proches en perte d'autonomie suite à une maladie, September, 2015)

33. Eunice E .Lee,Dn Sc ,RN ,Carol J.Farran Depression among Korean, Korean American and Caucasian American Family Journal of Transcultural Nursing,Vol15 N°1,2004,18-

25

34. Faiz et al, Strategy for the early management of ischemic stroke ANNALES DE MEDECINE ET DE THERAPEUTIQUE AMETHER.

October 2009; Volume 1, N° 1: 40 - 43

35. Fatoye FO, Komolafe MA, Adewuya AO, Fatoye GK.Emotional distress and self-reported quality of life among primary caregivers of stroke survivors in Nigeria.East Afr Med J. 2006 May; 83(5):271-9.

36. Forsberg-Warleby G, Moller A, Blomstrand C. Psychological well-being of spouses of stroke patients during the first year after stroke. Clin Rehabil. 2004; 18:430-7.

37. Gbiri CA, Olawale OA, Isaac SO.Stroke management: Informal caregivers' burdens and strains of caring for stroke survivors.Ann Phys Rehabil Med. 2015 Apr; 58(2):98-103. doi: 10.1016/j.rehab.2014.09.017. Epub 2015 Jan 7

38. Gosman-Hedström, G.; Claesson, L.; Blomstrand, C. (2008). Consequences of severity at stroke onset for health-related quality of life (HRQL) and informal care: a 1-year followup in elderly stroke survivors. Archives of gerontology and geriatrics. 47 (1) s. 79-91.

39. Grant, J.S., Weaver, M., Elliot, T.R., Bartolucci, A.R., & Newman, G.J. (2004). Sociodemographic, physical and psychosocial factors associated with depressive behaviour in family caregivers of stroke survivors in the acute care phase. Brain Injury, 18(8), 797-809.

40. Green, T.L., & King, K.M. (2007). The trajectory of minor stroke recovery for

men and their female spousal caregivers: Literature review. Journal of Advanced Nursing, 58(6), 517-531.

41.   Greenwood N, Mackenzie A.An exploratory study of anxiety in carers of stroke survivors.J Clin Nurs. 2010 Jul; 19(13-14):2032-8. doi: 10.1111/j.13652702.2009.03163.x.

42.   Hackett ML, Anderson CS. Predictors of Depression after Stroke A Systematic Review of Observational Studies. Stroke. 2005 Oct; 36(10):2296-301. PubMed Google Scholar

43.   Han B, Haley WE. Family caregiving for patients with stroke: review and analysis.

Stroke 1999;30:1478-85.

44.   HAS. Working together to improve stroke management practices

Cerebral. 2010 Review. www.has-sante.fr

45.   https://www.health-data-hub.fr/projets/le-vecu-des-proches-aidants-des-patients-victims-of-cerebral-vascular-accident-a

46.   Huybrechts KF, Caro JJ, Xenakis JJ, Vemmos KN. The prognostic value of the modified Rankin Scale score for long- term survival after first-ever stroke. Results from the Athens Stroke Registry.Cerebrovasc Dis. 2008; 26(4):381- 7.

47.   INESSS, L'organisation et la prestation des services de réadaptation pour les personnes ayant subi un AVC et leurs proches. Report written by Annie Tessier ETMIS 2012; 8(9): 1-101

48.   Jaracz K, Grabowska-Fudala B, Górna K, Jaracz J, Moczko J, Kozubski W. Burden in caregivers of long-term stroke survivors: Prevalence and determinants at months and 5 years after stroke. Patient Educ Couns. 2015 Aug; 98(8):1011-6. doi:

10.1016/j.pec.2015.04.008. Epub 2015 Apr 24.

49.   Jaracz K, Grabowska-Fudala B, Górna K, Kozubski W.Caregiving burden and its determinants in Polish caregivers of stroke survivors. Arch Med Sci. 2014 Oct

27; 10(5):941-50. doi: 10.5114/aoms.2014.46214. Epub 2014 Oct 23.

50. Jeanne Tyrrell L'épuisement des aidants familiaux: Facteurs de risque et réponses thérapeutiques Editions Chronique sociale,Lyon 2004

51. Jen Wen Himg and Sols Chrom g Ging Factors associated with Strain in informal caregivers of stroke patients. Med J2012, 35,392.

52. Kamel AA, Bond AE, Sivarajan Froelicher E Depression and caregiver burden experienced by caregivers of Jordanian patients with stroke. International Journal of
Nursing Practice 2012; 18: 147-154

53. Kessler et al, Generalized anxiety disorders,1994

54. Kintoki Fabien, Non-modifiable risk factors, el nino seasons and treatment, 2007

55. Krystyna Jaracz, Barbara Grabowska-Fudala, Krystyna Górna, Wojciech Kozubski Caregiving burden and its determinants in Polish caregivers of stroke survivors Arch Med Sci 5, October / 2014

56. Lalit Kalra, Andrew Evans et al. Training carers of stroke patient: Randomised controlled trial BMJ vol 328, 2014.

57. Langevin V,Francois M, Boini S Hospital Anxiety and Depression Scale Doc Med Trav.2011;125:23-35.

58. Lena Olai et al, Life situations and the care burden for stroke patients and their informal caregivers in a prospective cohort study,Upsala journal of Medical Sciences.2015.

59. M. Damak, I. Feki, M. Mezganni, C. Triki, N. Rekik and C. Mhiri. "Prognostic factors in acute-phase arterial stroke". RMNSCI.NET, Issue 1, November 19, 2006, http://www.rmnsci.info/ document. php?id=303.

60. M.P. Lindsay, G. Gubitz, M. Bayley, S. Phillips (editors), Canadian Best Practice Recommendations for Stroke Care) 4e edition, 2013

61. Magloire Nkosi Mpembi, Samuel Mampunza ma Miezi et al

Sociodemographic profile and social support for stroke depression in Kinshasa: A rehabilitation based crosssectional study, open Journal Of Epidemiology, 2013, 3,111-117

62. Manning L, Katbamna S, Johnson M et al British Indian carers of stroke survivors experience higher levels of anxiety and depression than White British carers: findings of a prospective observational study Diversity and Equality in Health and Care 2014;11:187-

200

63. Mapoure YN ; Kuate C, Bibaya et al. , Stroke costs at the General Referral Hospital of

Douala ;Health Sci Dis :Vol15 2014

64. Markey, E. (2015). The Impact of Caregiving on the Development of Major Depressive Disorder and Generalized Anxiety Disorder. Journal of European Psychology Students, 6(1), 17-24, DOI: http://dx.doi.org/10.5334/jeps.cn.

65. Mc Cullagh, E., Brigstocke, G., Donaldson, N., & Kalra, L. (2005). Determinants of caregiving burden and quality of life in caregivers of stroke patients. Stroke, 36, 21812186.

66. Mc Lennon SM, Bakas T, Jessup NM, Habermann B, Weaver MT. Task difficulty and life changes among stroke family caregivers: relationship to depressive symptoms. Arch Phys Med Rehabil. 2014 Dec; 95(12):2484- 90. doi:10.1016/j.apmr.2014.04.028. Epub 2014 May 22.

67. Mpembi M. N., Miezi S. M., Nzuzi T. M., et al. Clinical profile of post cerebrovascular depression: descriptive cross-sectional study in the rehabilitation center for people with disabilities of Kinshasa (DR Congo) The Pan African Medical Journal. 2014;17: p. 109. doi: 10.11604/pamj.2014.17.109.3296.

68. Nicolas Conde What are the issues faced by caregivers of patients in the sub-acute phase of a stroke?

? 2019 - 2020

69. Oladiji J. O., Akinbo S. R., Aina O. F., Aiyejusunle C. B. Risk factors of post-

stroke depression among stroke survivors in Lagos, Nigeria. African Journal of Psychiatry (Johannesbg) 2009;12(1):47-51.

70. Ostwald, S.K., Godwin, K.M., & Cron, S.G. (2009). Predictors of life satisfaction in stroke survivors and spousal caregivers twelve to twenty- four months post discharge from inpatient rehabilitation. Rehabilitation Nursing, 34(4), 160-174.

71. P. Antoine, S. Quandalle, V. Christophe. Living with a sick loved one: assessing the positive and negative dimensions of caregivers'experience. Annales Médico-

Psychologiques, Revue Psychiatrique, 2010, 168 (4), pp.273. ff10.1016/j.amp.2007.06.012ff. ffhal-00638570f

72. Perrocheau Ange Sophie, Return home for stroke patients: issues, limits, objectives, means 2015

73. Qurat UL Ain et Al Caregiver stress in stroke survivor data from a tertiary care a cross sectional survery Ain et Al,BMC Psychology 2014,2:49 htp "www.biomedcentral.com/2050-7283/49

74. Rapport d'activités 2011, CNSA (Caisse nationale de solidarité pour l'autonomie) April

2012

75. Rigby H, Gubitz G, Eskes G, et al. Caring for stroke survivors: baseline and 1-year determinants of caregiver burden. Int J Stroke 2009; 4:152-8.

76. Roopchand-Martin S, Creary-Yan S.Level of Caregiver Burden in Jamaican

77. Saban KL, Mathews HL, Bryant FB, O'Brien TE, Janusek LW.Depressive symptoms and diurnal salivary cortisol patterns among female caregivers of stroke survivors.Biol

Res Nurs. 2012 Oct; 14(4):396-404. Epub 2012 Apr 23

78. Selim Omrani Study of the quality of life of caregivers of elderly patients with cognitive disorders in memory consultation 2014.

79.   S Roopchand-Martin, S Creary-Yan Level of Caregiver Burden in Jamaican Stroke Caregivers and Relationship between Selected Sociodemographic Variables West Indian Med J. 2014 Jul 3; 63(6):605-9. doi: 10.7727/ wimj.2013. 060. Epub 2014 Jun 11.

80.   Sharon K. Ostwald et al, Stress experienced by stroke survivors and spousal caregivers during the first year after discharge from inpatient Rehabilitation Top Stroke Rehab.2009, 16(2):93-104

81.   Ski C, O'Connell B. Stroke: the increasing complexity of carer needs. J Neurosci Nurs 2007; 39:1729.

82.   Smith, L.N., Norrie, J., Kerr, S.M., Lawrence, I.M., Langhorne, P., & Lees, K.R. (2004). Impact and influences of caregiver outcomes at one year post-stroke. Cerebrovascular Diseases, 18(2), 145-153.

83.   Sognigbe N. Particularities of cerebrovascular accidents in Togo and sub-Saharan Africa. Thesis of medicine Lomé,Togo. 2006

84.   Taha S, Kazan RS. The meaning of caregiving experience lived by Lebanese family caregivers of stroke survivors at home Rech Soins Infirm. 2015 Mar;(120):88101.

85.   Tang WK, Lau CG, Mok V, Ungvari GS, Wong KS.Burden of Chinese stroke family caregivers: the Hong Kong experience.Arch Phys Med Rehabil. 2011 Sep; 92(9):1462-7. doi: 10.1016/j.apmr.2011.03.027.

86.   Tchokote, E. (2020). Experiences of family caregivers providing care to their parents with stroke in Cameroon: a phenomenological interpretive analysis. Nursing Research, 140, 97-106. https://doi.org/10.3917/rsi.140.0097

87.   Touzani, Stroke in Morocco Cerdi/Lasaare/2013

88.   UO Okoye, SS Asa Caregiving and Stress: Experience of People Taking Care of Elderly Relations in South-eastern Nigeria Arts and Social Sciences Journal, Volume 2011:

ASSJ-29

89.   Visser-Meily A, Van Heugten C,Post M, Schepers V, Lindeman

E,Intervention on Studies for caregivers of stroke survivors Patient education and Counseling 2005,56(3), 257-67.

90. Youssoufa Maiga, Mohamed Albakaye et al. Prise en charge des AVC au Mali (Afrique de l'Ouest) une enquête des pratiques Mali Medical 2013 Tome XXVIII, N°1,2010

91. Zahiruddin Othman, Siong Teck Wong, Ismail Drahman and Rahimah Zakaria.

Caregiver Burden is associated with cognitive Decline and Physical Disability of Elderly Post-Stroke Patient International Digital Organization for Scientific Information (IDOSI), 2014.

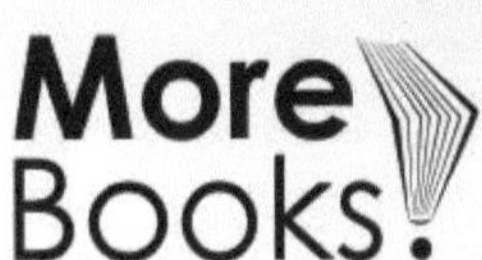

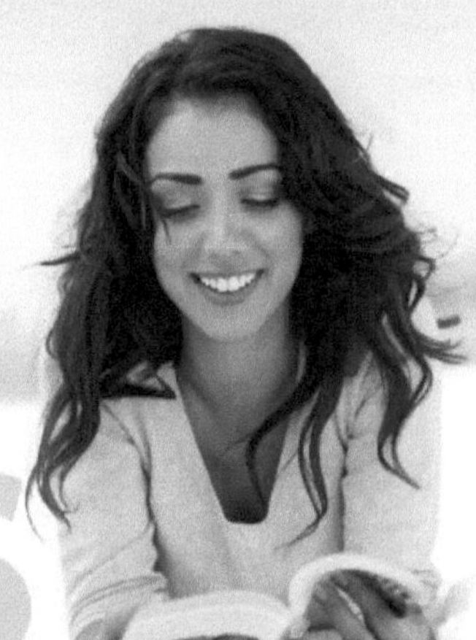

yes
I want morebooks!

Buy your books fast and straightforward online - at one of world's fastest growing online book stores! Environmentally sound due to Print-on-Demand technologies.

Buy your books online at
www.morebooks.shop

Kaufen Sie Ihre Bücher schnell und unkompliziert online – auf einer der am schnellsten wachsenden Buchhandelsplattformen weltweit! Dank Print-On-Demand umwelt- und ressourcenschonend produzi ert.

Bücher schneller online kaufen
www.morebooks.shop

info@omniscriptum.com
www.omniscriptum.com

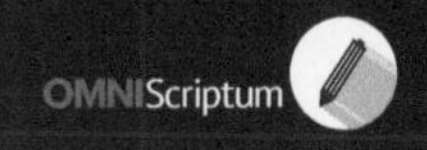

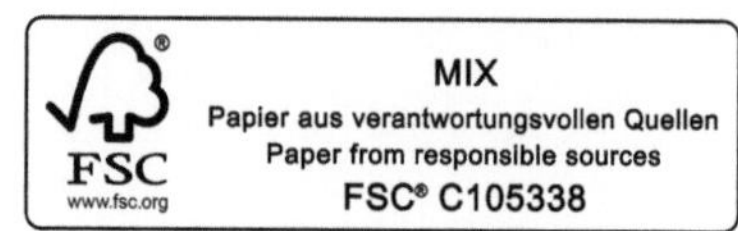

Printed by Books on Demand GmbH, Norderstedt / Germany